THE BEGINNER'S GUIDE TO

INTERMITTENT
KETO

THE BEGINNER'S GUIDE TO

INTERMITTENT KETO

Combine the Powers of
INTERMITTENT FASTING
with a **KETOGENIC DIET**
to Lose Weight and Feel Great

JENNIFER PERILLO

Little, Brown Spark
New York   Boston   London

Copyright © 2019 by Hachette Book Group

Hachette Book Group supports the right to free expression and the value of copyright. The purpose of copyright is to encourage writers and artists to produce the creative works that enrich our culture.

The scanning, uploading, and distribution of this book without permission is a theft of the author's intellectual property. If you would like permission to use material from the book (other than for review purposes), please contact permissions@hbgusa.com. Thank you for your support of the author's rights.

Little, Brown Spark
Hachette Book Group
1290 Avenue of the Americas, New York, NY 10104
littlebrownspark.com

First Edition: January 2019

Little Brown Spark is an imprint of Little, Brown and Company, a division of Hachette Book Group, Inc. The Little, Brown Spark name and logo are trademarks of Hachette Book Group, Inc.

The publisher is not responsible for websites (or their content) that are not owned by the publisher.

The Hachette Speakers Bureau provides a wide range of authors for speaking events. To find out more, go to hachettespeakersbureau.com or call (866) 376-6591.

ISBN: 978-0-316-45641-8
LCCN: 2018965115

Contents

PART I

AN INTRODUCTION TO INTERMITTENT FASTING AND THE KETO DIET

MAKING A CHANGE FOR BETTER HEALTH

We are what we eat. Sounds like a simple, straightforward statement, right? Let's take it one step further, though, and consider *how* we eat. Chances are you're looking to make a change if you're reading this book. Maybe the goal is weight loss, trying to lose those last stubborn ten pounds. Perhaps you're exploring changing your diet for preventive measures to put yourself on a better health track for the future.

Intermittent fasting and ketosis, also referred to as IF and Keto, are probably familiar or at least recognizable terms, since you bought this book in the first place. Unlike fad diets, where you might see fast results that are hard to maintain long term, both intermittent fasting and keto target the root systems of how you consume food and the choices you make with each meal. Implemented properly, intermittent fasting and keto are lifestyle changes, and long-term solutions for a healthier, happier you.

Today's availability of information means everything we want to know about anything is at our fingertips, or with a swipe of one. That same convenience can often leave you with an overload of information. How do you decipher it all and determine if intermittent fasting and keto are right for you? That's the goal of this book. I did a deep dive into both lifestyles and analyzed the benefits of both practices—implemented on their own and combined—so you can cut straight to the chase and get started on your intermittent keto journey.

Before you set out making changes, approach this as you would any recipe—read the directions from beginning to end first. Make sure you understand not just how to do intermittent fasting and cook keto-friendly meals but the science behind it all. Reading all the introductory material will make the transition to this new lifestyle easier and help you see the 4-Week Plan through to completion. Tempting as it might be to skip straight to the 4-Week Plan and recipes, keep in mind that a solid foundation is the key to success. The words between this introduction and the recipes provide the bricks and mortar to build a solid start.

Be prepared for the naysayers. We'll talk about this more in the Before You Get Started section on page 18. Everyone is an expert nowadays, ready to share their opinions whether welcome or not. Remember only YOU are an expert on you. One you've read through the following sections, you'll know if intermittent keto is right for you. Of course, if you have any underlying health concerns, always consult a medical practitioner before making any changes to your diet and lifestyle.

WHAT IS KETOSIS?

On the surface, carbohydrates are a quick, often fast and inexpensive form of nutrition to power through each day. Think about all those grab-and-go snacks we associate with breakfast—granola bars, fruit-filled smoothies, muffins. We start our mornings with carbs, and we keep piling them on as the day progresses.

Just because something works doesn't mean it's the most efficient means. The tissues and cells that make up our bodies need energy to perform everyday functions to keep us alive. There are two primary sources from which they can draw energy from the foods we eat. One form of energy is carbohydrates, which convert to glucose. That is the current model that most of us follow. There's an alternative fuel, though, and a surprising one: fat. Yes, the very thing you've been told to limit your entire life might just be the resource you need to jump-start your metabolism. Organic compounds, called ketones, are released when our bodies metabolize food and break down fatty acids. Ketones act as energy to keep our cells and muscles functioning.

You've likely heard the word "metabolism" throughout your life, but do you know what it means exactly? The term simply refers to the chemical reactions required in any living organism to stay alive. Of course, our metabolism is anything but simple given the complexities of the human body. Our bodies are constantly at work. Even when we're sleeping, our cells are continually building and repairing. They need to extract the energy from within our bodies.

Glucose, which is what carbs are broken down into once we eat them, is one way to fuel our metabolism. Our current nutrition guidelines focus on carbs as the primary source of energy. Factor in any additional sugars we eat and the recommended daily servings of fruit, starchy vegetables, grains, and plant-based forms of protein (e.g., beans), and there's no lack of glucose in our bodies. The problem with this model of energy consumption is that it leaves us like hamsters running on one of those wheels. We're burning energy but getting nowhere, especially if we're consuming more carbs than our bodies can use in a day's work.

But there's that other form of energy I mentioned: fat. How does that work exactly? Is it possible that tapping into that alternative fuel source will help our bodies burn energy more efficiently, with greater overall benefit to our health? We're back to that old idea of you are what you eat, except now think about the principal theory instead as you *burn* what you eat. That's where ketosis comes into play. Switching to a high-fat, moderate-protein, low-carb diet allows your body to enter a state of ketosis, wherein you metabolize fat, triggering a release of ketones to fuel the functions of our elaborate inner workings. The liver releases ketones after fatty acids are broken down.

Achieving a state of ketosis is about balance, but not the kind you're used to when it comes to eating. It turns out that our current food pyramid, which instructs us to consume an inordinate amount of carbohydrate-rich foods for energy, is upside down. A more efficient plan for fueling your body has fats at the top, making up 60 to 80 percent of your diet; protein in the middle at 20 to 30 percent; and carbs (really glucose in disguise) way at the bottom, accounting for just 5 to 10 percent of your daily eating plan.

KETO VS. PALEO

Evolution offers us many benefits. The ability to use fire and electricity to cook our food is proof alone that progress can be a good thing. Somewhere between our hunter-gatherer foraging lifestyle and today's modern world, a big disconnect happened. Sure, we have longer life spans now, but what about the quality of those extra years from a health perspective? The sluggish feeling that never seems to go away may be not just because you need to get extra sleep (though sleep is always a good thing!).

If food is fuel for our bodies, then it's safe to say that what we eat has an impact on our productivity. Put diesel in a car designed to run on gasoline and the effects are disastrous. Is it possible our bodies are in a similar state today, the result of our systems' having evolved to rely on carbs for energy as food became more reliably available, instead of fat, as in our early days of existence? I realize this sounds an awful lot like advocating for a paleo diet, but while the ketogenic lifestyle looks similar, the underlying principle to keto is vastly different. Keto is about creating a synergy between what you eat and the way your body functions—that's why the focus is on a specific manipulation of macronutrients (fat, protein, carbohydrates, fiber, and fluids). Every calorie is made up of specific macronutrients. Understanding why you're making such specific food choices is key to comprehending the bigger picture.

Fiber, for example, keeps us regular because it helps food pass through the digestive system. What goes in must come out, and fiber is essential to that process. Protein aids in tissue repair, producing enzymes and building bones, muscles, and skin. Fluids keep us hydrated—without them, our cells, tissues, and organs cannot function properly. Carbohydrates' primary role is to provide energy, but to do so, the body must convert them into glucose, which has a ripple effect throughout the rest of the body. Carb consumption is a delicate balance for people with diabetes because of its relationship to insulin production from increased blood sugar levels. Healthy fats support cell growth, protect our organs, help keep us warm, and have the ability to provide energy, but only when carbohydrates are consumed in limited quantities. I'll explain more about why and how that happens shortly.

CARBS VS. NET CARBS

Carbohydrates exist in some form in almost every food source. Total elimination of carbs is impossible and impractical. We need some carbohydrates to function. It's important to know this if we want to understand why some foods that fall into the restricted category on a keto diet are better choices than others.

Fiber counts as a carb in the nutritional breakdown of a meal. What's important to note is that fiber does not significantly affect our blood sugar—a good thing, since it's an essential macronutrient that helps us digest food properly. By subtracting the amount of fiber from the number of carbs in the nutritional tally of an ingredient or finished recipe, you're left with what's called net carbs.

Think about your paycheck before taxes (gross), and after (net). A terrible analogy, perhaps, since no one enjoys paying taxes, but an effective one in trying to understand carbs versus net carbs and how to track them. You put a certain number of carbs into your body, but not all of them affect your blood sugar level.

This doesn't mean you can go crazy with whole-grain pasta. Even though it's a better choice than white-flour pasta, overall, you should be limiting your net carbs to 20 to 25 grams per day. To put that in perspective: two ounces of uncooked whole-grain pasta have about 35 grams of carbohydrates and only 7 grams of total fiber. Probably pasta and bread are the two main things that people will ask you if you miss. Best way to answer them is by sharing all the things you *can* eat (see the Keto Cheat Sheet on page 30).

HOW LONG DOES IT TAKE FOR KETOSIS TO KICK IN?

Most people transition into ketosis within one to three days. It can take some people a full week, as all bodies are different. Factors that affect how quickly you enter ketosis include your current body weight, diet, and activity level.

In order to enter ketosis, your body needs to first burn through its glycogen (glucose) supply. Once the glycogens are depleted, your body signals it's time to start breaking down those fatty acids. During the next few days, the liver gets the message to begin excreting ketones. This last part of the process signals that you're in ketosis. The early stage is a mild ketosis, as ketone levels will be relatively low until you maintain ketosis for a steady period of time. You can measure ketone levels formally (see page 19), but you might start to notice some physiological changes that show you're in ketosis, such as keto flu or keto breath. They are not as severe or dramatic as they sound, and the benefits of ketosis might outweigh the downside in this phase-in period toward your defined goals, but it's good to familiarize yourself with the symptoms nonetheless (see pages 22 and 25).

INTERMITTENT FASTING: WHAT DOES IT MEAN?

When you say the phrase "Today I will fast," what is the first thing that comes to mind? Let me guess—is it "But I don't want to starve"? You're not alone in this common misconception, so let's break it down and make it easier to digest (pun very much intended!).

Fasting vs. Starvation

Fasting is a conscious choice. What sets fasting apart from starvation is that it's a decision you make to intentionally not eat. The length of time you choose to fast and the purpose for fasting (be it for religious reasons, weight loss, or a detox) are not forced upon you. Fasting is done at will. Done properly, fasting can have positive effects on our overall health.

Starvation is brought upon people unwillingly by a set of circumstances out of their control, famine, poverty, and war being just a few reasons for such a catastrophic situation. Starvation is a severe deficiency in calories that can lead to organ damage and eventually death. No one chooses to starve.

Once I thought about not eating from this perspective, it made perfect sense, and it was so much easier to wrap my head around the idea. Yes, at first I was skeptical about fasting too. Before I understood that there is a difference between fasting and starving, my first reaction to the idea of not eating was always "Why would anyone choose to starve?" The reality is, anyone who decides to fast is only choosing not to eat for a predetermined period of time. Even peaceful protests that use fasting as a means to an end have a defined goal for fasting.

Will You Feel Hungry While Fasting?

To answer that, let's put the question in perspective. The truth is, we all fast once a day. We often eat our last meal a few hours before going to sleep, and except for nursing newborns, I can't think of anyone who eats the moment they wake. Even if you average only six hours of sleep a night, it's likely you're already fasting ten hours a day. Now let's add the idea of intermittent to the mix. "Intermittent" means something that is not continuous. When applying that to the idea of fasting, it means you're lengthening the time when you don't eat between meals (the word "breakfast" means just that, breaking the fast).

Since our bodies are already accustomed to fasting once a day, the bigger issue is mind over matter. Let's get back to the question of whether you will feel hungry. The first week may be an adjustment as you get used to the extended period of time in your new fasting goal. To help you adjust, the 4-Week Intermittent Keto Plan on page 41 builds the fasting part of your day into your sleeping hours. It's quite possible your body will start to feel hungry around whatever time you're currently used to eating breakfast if it's before noon, but you will adjust within a few days.

In anticipation of the change you're about to make, try pushing back your first meal of the day by thirty minutes every day for a week before starting the 4-Week Plan. This way, when you begin the schedule laid out on page 42, you'll need to adjust your timing of your final meal of the day only once you begin week two of the plan for the Meals from Noon to 6 p.m. Only schedule.

Why Choose Intermittent Fasting?

Now that we've cleared up what it really means to fast, and you realize it's a conscious choice not to eat for a period of time, you might be still be wondering, why bother? The main reason that intermittent fasting (commonly referred to as IF) has taken the diet world by storm is its ability to promote weight loss. Metabolism is often categorized as one function of the human body. In reality, metabolism involves two essential reactions: catabolism and anabolism.

Catabolism is the part of metabolism wherein our bodies break down the food we consume. During catabolism, complex molecules are broken down into smaller units that release energy. Anabolism then uses that energy to begin the process of rebuilding and repairing our bodies, growing new cells, and maintaining tissues. Technically speaking, catabolism and anabolism happen simultaneously, but the rate at which they occur is different. A traditional eating schedule, where we spend the majority of our day eating, means our bodies have less time to spend in the second, or anabolic, phase of metabolism. It's a little confusing, perhaps, because the processes are interdependent, but remember that the rates at which they occur differ. The important takeaway here is that fasting for an elongated period allows for maximum efficiency in the metabolic processes.

Another amazing side effect of fasting, even for an intermittent period as outlined in this book, is a resurgence in mental acuity. Numerous studies show that contrary to popular belief, fasting makes you more aware and focused, not tired or light-headed. Many point to evolution and our ability to survive as a species: long before food preservation was possible, mental awareness was necessary at all times so that we could live from day to day, regardless of how plentiful food resources may have been.

Scientific research points toward neurogenesis, the

growth and development of nerve tissue in the brain, kicking into high gear during periods of fasting.

All roads lead toward one exceptionally important conclusion when it comes to fasting: it allows your body time to do more of the behind-the-scenes work necessary. The longer you extend the window between eating your last meal of one day and consuming the first meal of the following one, the more time your body must focus on cellular regeneration and tissue repair at all levels.

Are Liquids Allowed When Fasting?

There's one last important detail to note about intermittent fasting. Unlike religious fasting, which generally restricts consuming any food or liquids during the fast period, IF allows you to consume certain liquids. Technically speaking, the moment you consume anything with calories, a fast is broken. Looking at it through the lens of using intermittent fasting for its weight-loss benefits means we can apply different rules.

Bone broth (page 90) is recommended to replenish vitamins and minerals, and to maintain sodium levels. Coffee and tea are allowed, preferably without any added milk or cream, and with absolutely no sweeteners. There are two schools of thought on adding dairy to your coffee or tea. Provided it's only a high-fat addition, such as coconut oil or butter to make bulletproof coffee (page 87), many keto advocates think it's fine, since it doesn't disrupt ketosis. Adding MCT (medium-chain triglyceride) oil is believed to boost energy levels and leave you feeling sated as well. Purists adhere to plain coffee or tea. You should do what works best for you, provided it doesn't kick you out of ketosis (for ways to test for this, see pages 19–20).

Let's not forget water, as staying well hydrated is essential to any healthy lifestyle choices. Caffeine can be especially depleting, so make sure to balance coffee consumption with water intake too.

THE POWER OF INTERMITTENT FASTING & KETO COMBINED

By now, the benefits of intermittent fasting and adhering to a keto diet should be evident. What you might not have pieced together is the connection between the two. When you're in ketosis, that process of breaking down fatty acids to produce ketones for fuel is actually what the body does to keep itself going when you're fasting. What does it mean to combine the two, and why bother blending these lifestyles and ways of eating?

Fasting for one to two days has a significant effect when eating a traditional carb-centric diet. After the initial phase of burning glucose (that is, carbohydrates) for energy, your body naturally switches to burning fat as fuel.

You see where I'm going here, right? If it takes twenty-four to forty-eight hours for your body to switch to burning fat for fuel, imagine the effects of combining intermittent fasting with keto. Maintaining a constant state of ketosis means your body is already burning fat for fuel. This means the longer you spend in a state of fasting, the longer you're burning fat. Intermittent fasting combined with keto makes fasting's weight-loss effects more efficient, often resulting in more weight loss than traditional diets. The prolonged time between your last and first meals of the day means extra fat-burning capabilities for your body.

Ketosis is often used in body building because it's a safe way to shed fat without losing muscle. Weight loss is good only when it's the right weight, and we all need muscle mass to stay healthy.

How Does It Work?

Switching to the keto diet is a huge lifestyle change. For that reason, it's best to ease into the intermittent fasting aspect of this program. Let your body adjust to a new way of eating, get adapted to burning fat for fuel, and deal with any possible side effects (remember keto flu is a possibility) before incorporating intermittent fasting into your eating routine, or in this case, your extended period of not eating. Notice that intermittent fasting is not introduced until Week 2 of the 4-Week Plan.

During the phase-in period, you'll want to take note of eating times. Even before you incorporate the intermittent-fasting component of the plan, your last meal of the day should be no later than 6 p.m. This will ease you into fasting and help you avoid snacking. One of the effects of keto is that it trains your body—and, let's face it, your brain—to eat only when you're hungry. As times goes by, cravings cease. We often confuse cravings with hunger, when really cravings are a learned behavior, whereas hunger is a physiological call to refuel our energy reserves.

Timing Your Fasting Period

How you decide to incorporate your intermittent-fasting time is a bit flexible. Do you tend to dive into the water head first, or do you dip your toes in first? Knowing that about your personality will help you determine which schedule is better for you. In talking with my editor while writing this book, I learned that what was appealing to me was not to her.

I don't like feeling in a rut, and breakfast is one of my favorite meals of the day, so for me, having an alternate schedule that allows me to eat breakfast and abstain from dinner just about every other day, and to do the reverse on the other days (fasting through breakfast and eating dinner), is preferable. My editor, Marisa, prefers consistency, something I imagine a lot of people might want as well—to go on auto-pilot and fast at the same time every day. I can see how one or the other would fit into certain lifestyles and mind-sets, and that's why there are two schedules to choose from (pages 42–43). They allow you to customize the Intermittent Keto Plan to fit best with your lifestyle.

BEFORE YOU GET STARTED

Looking at the big picture is key to long-term success in any situation. This holds especially true for major diet and lifestyle changes. Intermittent keto throws everything you thought you knew about how to eat, what to eat, and when to eat it out the window. It's not a leap-without-looking kind of decision, so it's important to familiarize yourself with what to expect, how to handle potential challenges, and how to reorganize your life in a way that enables you to achieve your goals *before* starting out.

Define Your Goals

Why did you decide to try intermittent keto? Is it for health reasons? Weight loss? Are you looking just to feel better and increase your energy levels? Is this meant to be a short-term detox or are you looking to make long-term lifestyle changes? How do you plan to keep track of your macronutrients? Do you plan to test for ketones to ensure you've reached a state of ketosis? Are you vegetarian or vegan?

All are important questions to consider before getting started so you can stay focused on achieving your goal. Research suggests that intermittent fasting can have profound long-term benefits. The verdict is still out on the benefits or any potential risks of implementing a keto diet permanently. The rigidity of the plan also dictates the length of time people adhere to it.

The way you currently eat is also a big consideration

when you undertake keto, and you should understand how big a change or challenge that might pose. Keto is a fat-focused diet macronutrient-wise, but protein plays an important role. Too little protein can cause muscle loss during ketosis. Too much can kick you out of ketosis. It's a balance, and while keto is not a high-protein diet, the default protein is often meat because the plant-based protein alternatives typically touted are too high in carbs compared with their ratio of fiber and protein, specifically beans, including tofu (which is made from soybeans).

This doesn't mean it's impossible to stay vegetarian on keto, especially if you're an ovo-lacto vegetarian (okay with eating eggs and dairy). Nonmeat protein sources that are not legumes include eggs, nuts and seeds, and cheese. The recipes in this book are geared toward an omnivorous diet. Meat plays a role in many of the recipes. You'll need to customize your meal plan, supplementing it with recipes from outside sources. The rest of the information included in this book will be extremely helpful, and this applies to vegans, too. If you want to give intermittent keto a try with a vegan diet, it is not impossible, but it will require even more careful planning to make sure you don't kick yourself out of ketosis by choosing protein sources too high in carbs. Many of the recipes in this book will need adjusting for your dietary needs, as well.

Testing for ketosis can be done in three ways: urine test strips; a blood ketone test (with a meter similar to the kind used to test blood-glucose levels); and a breath test (different from keto breath, which is discussed separately). Urine tests are considered the least effective, but they are the least expensive, with blood meters considered the most accurate. They are also, as you might've guessed, the costliest.

The real question is do you need to test for ketones? If your goal is to lose weight, and the pounds are dropping, plus you feel good (well rested and energetic) after the initial few weeks, testing for ketosis might be a moot point. The more important consideration when it comes to counting numbers is monitoring what you're eating.

Macronutrients vs. Calories: Which Should You Count?

Tracking your macronutrients is different from counting just calories. On keto the emphasis is on monitoring the amount of fat, protein, and carbohydrates you consume — all macronutrients have a specific calorie count:

    1 gram of fat = 9 calories

    1 gram of protein = 4 calories

    1 gram of carbohydrate = 4 calories

Counting macronutrients sounds harder than it is. Really, it's just closer scrutiny of each calorie consumed. It's still necessary to get a baseline metabolic rate, also referred to as BMR, to determine how many calories you should eat for weight maintenance and weight loss (another reason why defining your goals is important).

All these macronutrients play a vital role in both your overall health and achieving and staying in ketosis, but the one that gets the most scrutiny on keto are carbohydrates because they result in glucose during metabolism which is the energy source you're trying to steer your body away from using. Some research shows the actual amount of total carbs one can consume per day on keto is 50 grams or fewer — which, depending on the fiber content, results in 20 to 35 net carbs per day. The lower you can get the net carbs down, the faster your body will go into ketosis and the easier it'll be to stay in it.

Keeping in mind that we're aiming for 20 grams of net carbs a day, the fat and protein grams are variables depending on how many calories you need to consume based on your BMR. The recommended daily average for women varies between 1,600 and 2,000 calories for weight maintenance depending on level of activity (from sedentary to active). Adhering to a daily plan of consuming 160 grams fat + 70 grams protein + 20 grams carbohydrates mirrors 1,800 calories of eating — the ideal amount according to the USDA for weight maintenance for moderately active women (walking 1.5 to 3 miles a day). If you have a sedentary lifestyle — defined as getting exercise from such normal everyday activities as cleaning and walking short distances only — you'd want to aim for 130 grams fat + 60 grams protein + 20 grams carbohydrates to jump-start weight loss (1500 calories). There are plenty of online calculators to figure out your BMR and overall calorie goal, and to determine the right ratio of fat and protein, while keeping net carbs to 20 grams per day.

Speaking of calculators and tracking numbers, you might find it helpful to establish a tracking method for your macronutrients from the recipes in this book to help customize your own unique menu. It can be as easy as writing it down in a notebook and doing the math, but that might be more time consuming. There's no shortage of apps for your phone to also make easy work of tracking macronutrients.

THE PHYSICAL SIDE EFFECTS OF KETO

Unlike diet plans that simply limit the foods you eat for weight loss, keto goes deeper. Ketosis is about changing the way you eat to change the way your body converts what you eat into energy. The process of ketosis flips the equation from burning glucose (remember, carbs) to instead burning fat for fuel. This comes with possible side effects as your body adjusts to a new way of functioning. This is also why the 4-Week Plan on page 42 phases in intermittent fasting during week two, and not from the get-go. It's important to give yourself time, both physically and mentally, to properly transition. Two physical changes you may experience when transitioning to a keto diet are keto flu and keto breath.

Keto Flu

Keto flu, sometimes called carb flu, can last anywhere from a few days to a few weeks. Metabolic changes happening within as your body weans itself from burning glucose for energy may result in heightened feelings of lethargy, irritability, muscle soreness, light-headedness or brain fog, change in bowel movements, nausea, stomachaches, and trouble focusing and concentrating. I know, it sounds terrible, and probably vaguely familiar. Yes, these are all common symptoms of the flu, hence the name.

The good news is this is a temporary phase as your body adjusts, and it doesn't affect everyone. Factors causing these symptoms include an imbalance of electrolytes (sodium, potassium, magnesium, and calcium) and sugar withdrawal from the significantly decreased carbohydrate consumption. Expecting these possible symptoms means you can be prepared to alleviate them and decrease the length of keto flu, should it occur at all.

Sodium levels are directly affected by the amount of highly processed foods you consume. To clarify, everything we eat is technically a processed food; the term means "a series of steps performed to achieve a particular end." Even cooking at home from scratch requires the act of processing food. Relating to our current culture, though, where ready-to-eat foods are at every turn of the supermarket, these highly processed foods tend to contain exorbitant levels of hidden salt (sodium is a preservative as well as a flavor enhancer).

Adhering to a keto diet is most successful when you're doing the actual cooking, and you can control the number of carbs and amount of sugars in a dish. Home cooking tends to be less processed, which might also result in lower sodium. Increasing the amount of salt in your food and drinking a homemade stock such as the bone broth on page 90 are easy, natural ways to boost your sodium levels.

Below are other foods to focus on during your keto phase-in period. They're naturally rich in magnesium, potassium, and calcium to help keep your electrolytes in balance.

Magnesium (helps with muscle soreness and leg cramps)

Avocados, broccoli, fish, kale, almonds, pumpkin seeds, spinach

Potassium (helps with muscle soreness, hydration)

Asparagus, avocados, Brussels sprouts, salmon, tomatoes, leafy greens

Calcium (especially important if you were a big milk drinker pre-keto)

Almonds, bok choy, broccoli, cheese, collard greens, spinach, sardines, sesame and chia seeds

Another way to lessen the chances of experiencing keto flu is to begin slowly decreasing your carb intake a few weeks before starting the 4-Week Plan. It can be as simple as swapping your morning muffin for a hard-boiled or scrambled egg, skipping the bun and wrapping your burger in lettuce (often referred to as protein-style when ordering), or swapping out spaghetti for zoodles. This way, when you dive into the plan on page 42 or page 43, it'll feel more like a natural progression in eating fewer carbs than a sharp right turn in your diet.

Keto Breath

Let's cut to the chase here. Bad breath stinks, literally, but it's something you should brace yourself for when switching to keto. There are two thoughts as to why this occurs.

As your body enters ketosis and begins releasing ketones (a by-product of burning fat for fuel), one of the ketones released is acetone (yes, the same solvent found in nail polish remover and paint thinners). Acetone is excreted through urine and from your breath in the body's attempt to finish the metabolic process of breaking down those fatty acids. This can result in unpleasant-smelling breath.

Protein can also be a factor in contributing to keto breath. Remember, the macronutrient goal is high fat, moderate protein, and low carb. People often think high fat is interchangeable with high protein. That is far from true. The body digests fat and protein differently. Our bodies produce ammonia when breaking down protein and usually release it during urine output. Eating more protein than you need results in the indigestible amount lingering in your gut system, where it ferments, producing ammonia, which is then released through your breath.

The upside is that keto breath is a good indicator your body is in ketosis. How long the smell lasts varies according to how well your body adapts to ketosis. Many sources indicate it lasts anywhere from one week to just under a month. A deeper dig through keto message boards and chat groups shows it can persist for months, while some people report never experiencing it. Some solutions to possibly avoid or lessen keto breath are to always be armed with sugar-free gum, reduce your protein intake, make sure you stick to a good dental routine (brushing and flossing), and follow the advice mentioned earlier on gradually reducing your carbohydrate intake before jumping full steam ahead into the 4-Week Plan.

SLEEP & EXERCISE

Every healthy lifestyle includes adequate sleep and moderate activity. The same advice should be considered when defining your goals and figuring out how both fit into your daily routine. Once you incorporate intermittent fasting into your plan, those sleeping hours become even more necessary since they're part of your fasting time. Keep late-night snacking urges at bay by tucking in at a reasonable hour.

Weight training is a big focus among keto enthusiasts, and it's certainly important when you're in maintenance mode. When it comes to weight loss, cardio workouts provide the biggest fat-burning benefit. Be sure to consult your doctor before making any major changes if you have underlying health concerns.

TALK WITH YOUR FRIENDS & FAMILY

Mention the word "diet" and you'll find most people have strong opinions that increase in intensity with certain diet plans. Everyone is entitled to their opinions, and sharing similar experiences is sometimes helpful when you're looking for inspiration or motivation. What's not beneficial is when people say, "You look fine the way you are" or "I could never give up carbs" or, worse, "You're going to starve yourself?!"

Every ship needs a helmsman, so consider yourself the helmsman of your body. Friends and family should be there to support you on this journey, so empower them with the information to do so. Let them know why you're making the switch if you're comfortable talking about it. At the least, explain the principles behind why intermittent fasting and keto work really well for some people. Often people are simply confused by what they don't know, and they don't take the time to seek out answers. You can even give them a copy of this book if they want to look deeper into the diet. You never know if you'll inspire someone to want to try intermittent keto, too, and then you'll have a buddy to track progress, set goals with, and keep each other motivated.

Sharing your decision to go on keto is also a good way to avoid showing up at a friend's dinner party and discovering they're serving pasta only. In a circumstance like that, you should volunteer to bring a course to share that's also keto-friendly for you to enjoy. This way it alleviates any stress your host might feel about cooking for you, plus it highlights some of the amazing foods you can eat on keto!

There will be those who think they know better or insist it's okay to cheat here and there. Maybe that works for other diets, but you can easily knock yourself out of ketosis by consuming too many carbohydrates. Be a good advocate for yourself, and don't be afraid to say no thank you. People who care about you will respect the hard work you're putting into developing a healthier lifestyle for yourself and won't try to tempt you.

Obviously, you also want to keep your intermittent fasting schedule in mind when you're making plans. Late-night dinners don't really jibe with the plan, but you can meet for drinks and keep your order to plain seltzer with a lime wedge, or better yet meet for a post-dinner coffee. The 4-Week Plan was designed to give you a break from intermittent fasting on Sunday mornings, keeping in mind that's a popular time to gather with friends, and brunch is very easy to stick to on the keto diet.

STAYING IN KETOSIS & WHAT HAPPENS IF YOU FALL OUT OF IT

Once you enter ketosis, how long you decide to stick with it is up to you after you finish the 4-Week Plan. Was your goal simply to drop a dress size? A month may be all you need. Were you trying to wean yourself off sugar or reduce your overall carb intake? Perhaps a little longer might be good to help establish long-term eating patterns even after you decide to increase your total carb count beyond the 20 grams per day allotted in the 4-Week Plan. Technically anything less than 50 grams of carbohydrates (overall, not net carbs) helps kick your body into fat-burning mode, so even a minor increase in carbs can offer a mild ketosis benefit, though you might regain a few of the pounds you initially lost.

Be prepared for learning curves and possible pitfalls. It's

possible to kick your body out of ketosis if you eat too much protein, too many carbs, or don't get enough exercise. A simple mistake, or just giving into a craving such as eating a sweet potato, can put you back into glucose-burning mode.

If keto sounds strict, that's because it is. Getting into ketosis and maintaining it is a commitment—that's why we talked about defining your goals early on. While it might seem disastrous or frustrating after all the hard work you put in, don't beat yourself up. Focus on your future goals and on getting yourself back into ketosis. Don't extend the cheat, thinking, "Oh, well, the damage is done." Instead, fasting after a cheat day is one way to get yourself back on track, keeping in mind you'll have to burn through that glucose again first.

Journaling, in general, is a great way to track more than just calories. Start recording how you're feeling physically, and what your mental outlook is—a simple number rating system helps you understand if you're making progress, maintaining the status quo, or slipping with your goals. Detailed notes might help pinpoint more direct reasons related to your cheat day to help plan better in the future. In fact, it might be the case that you want to pad in cheat days so you can expect them, instead of beating yourself up for having them. If you know your best friend's wedding is coming up and you'll want to partake 100 percent in the festivities, including all the food and drink served, plan for that. While you can't just flip a switch to get back into ketosis, you'll know what to expect and hopefully get back on track quicker than the first time. It's also worth mentioning that you shouldn't rely on too many cheat days. Again, this goes back to defining your goals.

KNOW WHAT FOODS TO ENJOY & WHAT FOODS TO AVOID

It's so easy to think about what you can't eat on keto, but it's much more fun to focus on all the things you *can* enjoy. Here's a chart you can reference when you're in need of some inspiration.

KETO CHEAT SHEET

Eat	Avoid
Zoodles, spaghetti squash and shirataki noodles	Pasta
Use almond flour, unsweetened coconut flakes and pork cracklings	Bread crumbs
Cauliflower rice, shirataki rice	Rice, couscous
Heavy cream and cheeses (mozzarella, cheddar)	Milk
Low-carb tortillas and keto bread (page 92)	Bread, wraps, tortillas
Puréed cauliflower	Mashed potatoes
Zucchini fries	French fries and sweet potato fries
Berries; use lemons and limes for flavor	Sweet citrus (oranges, grapefruit, clementines), tropical fruits (bananas, mango, pineapple), all dried fruits
Meat, poultry, seafood, eggs	Beans, tofu
Stevia, monk fruit	Sweeteners (honey, maple syrup, sugar)
Olive oil, coconut oil, avocado oil, butter, ghee, sesame oil (in small quantities)	Sunflower, grapeseed, canola, peanut, safflower oils, margarine, vegetable shortening
Parmesan Crisps (page 97)	Chips and sweet/salty snacks
Water (key for staying hydrated), coffee, tea	Sugary drinks (soda, juices), alcohol

The Keto Kitchen

Leading up to starting intermittent keto, it's important to make sure your pantry aligns with your new eating goals. Those new goals might also be at odds with the rest of the members in your household, be they family or roommates. If so, clearing out all the carb-laden foods, sugary snacks, and processed foods might not be a possibility. In that case, it'll be an exercise in self-control for you, especially during the first week or two, when cravings might be tricky to manage. Don't fret. You can still claim an area of the kitchen and set up a keto-friendly zone to make sticking to the plan easier. And by all means, if you live on your own, or if your partner/family is doing this with you, go full throttle and use an out-with-the-old, in-with-the-new approach. Instead of discarding unwanted items, donate them to a local food pantry (check expiration dates first), or give them to your neighbors.

Once you've got a clean slate, it's time to start filling the pantry with all the foods you can enjoy. Here are staple ingredients you'll want to add to your first shopping list.

Fermented foods (make sure veggies are lacto-fermented): pickles, kimchi, sauerkraut, plain full-fat yogurt

Oils: avocado oil, extra virgin olive oil, cold-pressed or virgin coconut oil, ghee, MCT oil

Nuts and seeds (and flours made from them): almonds, walnuts, macadamia nuts, brazil nuts, pecans, chia seeds, pumpkin seeds, sunflower seeds, sesame seeds, almond flour or meal, coconut flour

Canned goods and other shelf-stable items (make sure all nut milks are unsweetened): coconut cream, coconut milk, almond milk, olives, dark chocolate (Lily's dark chocolate chips are sweetened with stevia), cocoa powder, tea and coffee (plain, unflavored), pork rinds, baking powder (see note below)

Spices and sweeteners: red pepper flakes, basil, oregano, bay leaves, smoked paprika, sea salts, black pepper, cumin, curry powder, everything-bagel seasoning, whole-grain mustard, stevia, monk fruit sweetener (read the label to make sure it's not a blend mixed with sugar)

Perishables: bacon and sausage (be sure to buy sugar-free varieties), eggs, coconut wraps, low-carb tortillas, sugar-free mayonnaise, heavy cream, butter, cheese

A Word About Baking Powder & Other Ingredients

One look at the ingredients and you'll notice there's cornstarch in commercial baking powder. It's actually in most homemade recipes, too. Baking powder is traditionally made with a combination of baking soda, cream of tartar, and cornstarch. Some keto folks will tell you cornstarch is absolutely forbidden, since it's a grain and you're not supposed to eat any grains on keto. It's important to remember why you're not supposed to eat grains, though, before settling on a conclusion about baking powder. The underlying reason is that grains are carb heavy, and keto is a low-carb diet. The reality is, the amount of cornstarch in baking powder compared with how much you actually use in a recipe is so negligible that it barely registers. If you're grain free for health reasons, that's a good reason to make your own baking powder or seek out a brand without any cornstarch. I've yet to find one that exists, but that may change by the printing of this book. All the recipes in this book were tested using store-bought baking powder. Results using a homemade version without cornstarch aren't guaranteed.

Most bacon has sugar added during the curing process, even bacon from small, artisanal farmers. While the actual amount of sugar in the end product is minimal, you might want to look for a brand that has no sugar added if you're having trouble balancing your carb count.

Not all ketchups are created equal. In fact, many are loaded with sugar. Be sure to buy an unsweetened brand like Primal Kitchen for dipping and to make the BBQ sauce on page 68.

Many keto enthusiasts swear by MCT oil. It's not coconut oil, but rather a by-product of coconut. MCT stands for medium chain triglycerides. Among the health benefits it is said to offer are that it keeps you satiated (feeling full), provides a quick boost of energy, and supports a healthy immune system. The full feeling it offers may be why some people believe it aids in weight loss, in that it prevents you from overeating or snacking.

Weekly Grocery Shopping

When it comes to produce, all herbs get a green light— great news, since they're easy flavor boosters to any meal. The general rule of thumb for vegetables is that you should stick to ones that grow aboveground. That means steer clear of root vegetables and tubers (think carrots, parsnips, beets, onions, and regular and sweet potatoes), as they're starchier vegetables, higher in carbohydrates. Some aboveground vegetables are high-carb, too, such as winter squash, pumpkin, corn, and peas.

You can still eat the rainbow, so don't worry—dark, leafy greens (kale, spinach), broccoli, cauliflower, zucchini (zoodles!), radishes, cucumbers, garlic, asparagus, mushrooms, and eggplant all make the list for keto meals.

Fruit lovers might find keto challenging, since most fruits are too high in natural sugars and therefore off-limits, especially dried fruits—which have higher concentrations of sugar. Your choices are basically berries (since they're mostly fiber), lemon, and limes. All other citrus fruits are too high in natural sugars. But guess what? If you love an orange essence in some dishes, you can use orange zest to add flavor without getting any of the carbs!

At this point, you might feel weighed down by all the things you can't eat. That's a normal feeling, and while it's a reality if you're committed to keto, I always prefer to focus on the foods you *can* eat, so snap a photo of that Keto Cheat Sheet on page 30, and you'll always have a quick reference point when in doubt.

Essential Kitchen Tools

Veteran cooks likely have a well-stocked kitchen. If you're just starting out, you'll quickly realize that cooking your own food increases your success in sticking to a keto diet. I tend to stay away from gadgets that serve only one purpose, but exceptions to that rule are my spiralizer and avocado slicer. Homemade zoodles are a breeze to make with my handheld spiralizer, found in the hardware store's kitchen section for less than $20.

Avocados are a keto fan-favorite. Pitting avocados also results in more emergency-room visits than you might imagine and can even result in nerve damage. This happened to a dear friend of mine who's an experienced cook. She now owns an avocado slicer.

Regarding skillets, I find nonstick to be great if you can buy only one set of pans. Even though you'll be consuming considerably more fat than you do in your current diet, nonstick skillets are great for making eggs and pancakes (check out the Blueberry Almond Pancakes on page 49).

Here's a list of kitchen tools and equipment that you'll find helpful in preparing meals:

8-inch skillet

10-inch skillet

Spiralizer

Digital kitchen scale

Bento box for packing lunches

Tongs and spatula

Avocado slicer

Mason jars (for preparing and transporting chia puddings)

Silicon candy molds (for making fat bombs)

Chef's knife and paring knife

Variety of saucepans (ranging from 2 quarts to 8 quarts, if space and budget permit)

Cutting boards

Blender

Food processor (optional, but especially helpful to grind your own nut flours)

WHEN TO STOP & HOW TO STOP

Keto is strict about what you can and cannot eat. Throw in intermittent fasting and you further restrict when you can eat. Before you dive into your 4-Week Plan, this is a good time to talk about how long you should stay on keto and continue your intermittent fasting. Currently there isn't enough research to make a conclusion from a health perspective as to keto's long-term efficacy, but the truth is you're fighting your body's natural instinct to fuel itself on glucose. Even though we evolved under the premise of fat for fuel, times have changed, and along with that, so have our bodies—for better or for worse.

Although research providing concrete theories of how the keto diet works (besides those related to underlying medical issues) is lacking, many people lean toward using keto a few times a year for a prolonged period of time—anywhere from a few weeks to a couple of months—taking a break in between but still being mindful of overall carb consumption.

Intermittent fasting is a different story. I know someone who's been fasting intermittently for a few years now. Her approach is different from the plan outlined here, and she is not on keto, so her experience is different, but intermittent fasting has been very successful and manageable for her to maintain. She's also one of the biggest foodies and cooks I know, and intermittent fasting hasn't cramped her style one bit. Quite the opposite, in fact. She looks forward to her fast days, as they leave her feeling refreshed and focused. Should you decide to step away from the keto diet and stay with intermittent fasting, I suggest doing some research to figure out the best method and schedule for yourself.

When you feel you've reached the end of your keto journey or just want to press pause for a duration beyond a cheat, you must do it in a meaningful and methodical way. Remember that it took time for your body to adjust to ketosis. The same goes for reverting to a diet that has more carbohydrates, which will flip the switch back to burning glucose for energy. This applies even if your plan is to stay on a lower-carb diet than you ate before starting keto.

Things to keep in mind when you decide to switch off keto are:

- Take it slowly, introducing more carbs a little at a time.
- Expect some weight gain. The amount depends on how long you've been on keto. The early weeks of weight loss on keto tend to be water weight. If you've been on keto for a while, the weight gain should be less, provided you're not overindulging in carbs and sugar.
- Familiarize yourself with healthy portion sizes again, adjusting the quality of fats and proteins accordingly.

PART II

MEAL PLANS AND RECIPES

READY, SET, GO: 4-WEEK PLANS & RECIPES

MEAL PLANS

The Weekend Before

Saturday. Clean out the pantry. Make shopping lists.
Sunday. Go grocery shopping—stick to the perimeter; all the super-processed items tend to be clustered in the middle aisles. Prep food for the week ahead.

4-WEEK PLAN — MEALS FROM NOON TO 6 P.M. ONLY

This plan allows for one day a week without fasting. It anticipates that you might want to enjoy a Sunday brunch with friends (keto foods only). If you want, you can omit breakfast to stick with your IF routine. Just be sure to include a midday snack to make sure you consume your necessary macronutrients.

Week 1	MON	TUES	WED	THUR	FRI	SAT	SUN
Morning	KETO	KETO	KETO	KETO	KETO	KETO	KETO
Noon	KETO	KETO	KETO	KETO	KETO	KETO	KETO
Pre 6pm	KETO	KETO	KETO	KETO	KETO	KETO	KETO
Week 2							
Morning	FAST	FAST	FAST	FAST	FAST	FAST	KETO
Noon	KETO	KETO	KETO	KETO	KETO	KETO	KETO
Snack	KETO	KETO	KETO	KETO	KETO	KETO	none
Pre 6pm	KETO	KETO	KETO	KETO	KETO	KETO	KETO
Week 3							
Morning	FAST	FAST	FAST	FAST	FAST	FAST	KETO
Noon	KETO	KETO	KETO	KETO	KETO	KETO	KETO
Snack	KETO	KETO	KETO	KETO	KETO	KETO	none
Pre 6pm	KETO	KETO	KETO	KETO	KETO	KETO	KETO
Week 4							
Morning	FAST	FAST	FAST	FAST	FAST	FAST	KETO
Noon	KETO	KETO	KETO	KETO	KETO	KETO	KETO
Snack	KETO	KETO	KETO	KETO	KETO	KETO	none
Pre 6pm	KETO	KETO	KETO	KETO	KETO	KETO	KETO

4-WEEK PLAN — ALTERNATE INTERMITTENT FASTING

Week 1	**MON**	**TUES**	**WED**	**THUR**	**FRI**	**SAT**	**SUN**
Morning	KETO	KETO	KETO	KETO	KETO	KETO	KETO
Noon	KETO	KETO	KETO	KETO	KETO	KETO	KETO
Pre 6pm	KETO	KETO	KETO	KETO	KETO	KETO	KETO
Week 2							
Morning	KETO	KETO	FAST	KETO	FAST	KETO	KETO
Noon	KETO	KETO	KETO	KETO	KETO	KETO	KETO
Pre 6pm	FAST	FAST	KETO	FAST	KETO	KETO	FAST
Week 3							
Morning	FAST	KETO	FAST	KETO	FAST	KETO	KETO
Noon	KETO	KETO	KETO	KETO	KETO	KETO	KETO
Pre 6pm	KETO	FAST	KETO	FAST	KETO	KETO	FAST
Week 4							
Morning	FAST	KETO	FAST	KETO	FAST	KETO	KETO
Noon	KETO	KETO	KETO	KETO	KETO	KETO	KETO
Pre 6pm	KETO	FAST	KETO	FAST	KETO	KETO	FAST

RECIPES

Cookbooks are generally broken into traditional categories of breakfast, lunch, dinner, and sweets and snacks. You'll find the recipes set up that way for familiarity. Since keto is all about focusing on your macronutrients, what really matters is eating the right ratios of fat, protein, and carbs. Keeping that in mind, feel free to swap out breakfast for lunch, lunch for dinner, or even dinner for breakfast. Just track your macros to make sure you don't overeat any of them.

BREAKFAST

Pecan & Coconut 'n' Oatmeal

Bacon, Egg & Cheese Breakfast "Muffins"

Cheddar Chive Baked Avocado Eggs

Blueberry Almond Pancakes

Toad in a Hole

Berry Breakfast Shake

Cheddar, Spinach & Mushroom Omelet

Pecan & Coconut 'n' Oatmeal

Serves: 1

This is a hearty breakfast porridge for cold mornings when you're craving a steaming bowl of oatmeal but don't want the carb overload.

- ½ cup coconut or almond milk
- 2 teaspoons chia seeds
- 2 tablespoons almond flour
- 1 tablespoon flax meal
- 2 tablespoons hemp hearts
- ¼ teaspoon ground cinnamon
- ¼ teaspoon pure vanilla extract
- 1 tablespoon pecans, toasted and chopped
- 1 tablespoon coconut flakes

In a small pot, combine the milk, chia seeds, almond flour, flax meal, hemp hearts, cinnamon, and vanilla. Cook over low heat, stirring constantly until thickened, about 5 minutes. Spoon into a bowl, top with the pecans and coconut flakes, and enjoy immediately.

Calories 312   Fat 25   Protein 13.4   Carbs 7   Fiber 5   Net carbs 2

BACON, EGG & CHEESE BREAKFAST "MUFFINS"

Makes: 6

- 6 slices bacon
- 8 eggs
- ¼ cup heavy cream
- Fine sea salt and freshly ground black pepper to taste
- 3 ounces shredded cheddar cheese

Preheat the oven to 375°F. Generously grease the bottoms and sides of a 6-cup muffin tin (softened butter works best for this).

Add the bacon to a cold 10-inch skillet, and place over medium-high heat. Cook until crisp all over, turning once. Transfer to a paper-towel line plate. Crumble the bacon into pieces.

In a deep bowl, whisk together the eggs, cream, salt, and pepper.

Sprinkle an even amount of cheese and bacon into each cup of the prepared tin. Pour an even amount of egg mixture over the filling.

Bake 20 to 25 minutes, until the eggs puff up and are lightly golden.

Calories 303   Fat 26   Protein 15   Carbs 1.5   Fiber 0   Net carbs 1.5

CHEDDAR CHIVE BAKED AVOCADO EGGS

Serves: 2

- 2 eggs
- 2 ounces cheddar cheese, shredded
- 2 teaspoons heavy cream
- 1 teaspoon fresh chopped chives
- Sea salt and freshly ground black pepper to taste
- 1 avocado, cut in half and pitted (see note)

Preheat the oven to 425F°.

Combine the eggs, cheddar cheese, cream, half the chives, salt, and pepper in a medium bowl. Beat with a fork until well mixed.

Arrange the avocados in a small rimmed baking dish, cut side up (they should be snug so they don't roll around). Pour the egg filling into the center of each avocado.

Bake 12 minutes, until the filling is lightly golden on top. Serve hot, topped with the remaining chives.

Note: Avocado pits vary, so depending on the size, you might need to scoop a little bit extra avocado from the center with a spoon to accommodate the egg filling.

Calories 257   Fat 22   Protein 13   Carbs 1.3   Fiber 0   Net carbs 1.3

BLUEBERRY ALMOND PANCAKES

Makes: 10 (serving size 2 pancakes)

Aside from the lack of grains, these pancakes are different from the usual in another way: you cover the pan with a lid while they're cooking to ensure that they cook through in the center.

- 4 tablespoons butter
- 2 large eggs
- ¼ cup almond milk
- ¼ teaspoon pure vanilla extract
- ¾ cup almond flour
- 1 tablespoon flax meal
- 1 teaspoon baking powder
- 1 packet stevia powder
- ¼ teaspoon sea salt
- ¼ teaspoon allspice (optional)
- ¾ cup blueberries, frozen or fresh
- Butter, to cook the pancakes

In a small bowl, whisk the butter, eggs, almond milk, and vanilla. Whisk in the flour, flax meal, baking powder, stevia, salt, and allspice until well blended. Fold in the blueberries.

Heat a nonstick skillet over medium heat. It's ready to use when a few drops of water dance across the surface. Melt a pat of butter in the pan. Drop scant ¼ cupfuls of batter into the skillet, spreading out into thin circles (they'll puff up). Cover the pan with a lid and cook 1 to 2 minutes until air bubbles appear on top and batter looks a little dry. Flip, and cook until cooked through and golden underneath, about 2 minutes more. Serve hot.

Note: Leftover pancakes may be layered between parchment paper, wrapped in plastic film and stored in the freezer for up to 1 month. Heat them straight from the freezer in a 350°F oven for 8 to 10 minutes.

Calories 114   Fat 10   Protein 3.9   Carbs 3.9   Fiber 1.4   Net carbs 2.5

TOAD IN A HOLE

Serves: 2

- 4 pork sausages (spicy or sweet)
- ⅓ cup blanched, fine almond flour
- 3 tablespoons arrowroot
- 6 tablespoons almond milk
- ¼ cup heavy cream
- 1 egg
- ¼ teaspoon sea salt

Place an 8-inch cast-iron skillet on the center rack of the oven. Preheat oven to 400F°.

Add the sausages to the skillet. Cook, turning once, until nicely browned, 12 to 15 minutes.

Meanwhile, combine the almond flour, arrowroot, almond milk, cream, egg, and salt in a medium bowl. Whisk until mixed well.

Once the sausages are browned, pour the batter into the hot pan. Return the skillet to the oven, and cook until puffed up and golden, 20 to 25 minutes. Serve immediately.

Calories 376   Fat 28   Protein 16.3   Carbs 16.2   Fiber 2.4   Net carbs 13.8

BERRY BREAKFAST SHAKE

Serves: 1

- ¼ cup frozen mixed berries
- ½ cup heavy cream
- ½ cup coconut or almond milk
- 1 tablespoon almond butter
- ½ teaspoon fresh squeezed lemon juice
- 1 tablespoon MCT oil (optional)

Add all the ingredients to a blender bowl. Blend until smooth. Serve immediately.

Calories 900   Fat 80   Protein 10   Carbs 18   Fiber 5   Net carbs 13

Cheddar, Spinach & Mushroom Omelet

Serves: 2

Sure, this is included in the breakfast category, but omelets are also a great go-to meal for lunch and dinner, so keep this recipe in mind when planning your menu for the week.

- 2 teaspoons extra virgin olive oil
- 3 ounces white button mushrooms, sliced
- 2 cups packed baby spinach
- Sea salt, to taste
- Handful of fresh parsley, chopped
- 6 large eggs, lightly beaten
- 4 ounces cheddar cheese, shredded

In an 8-inch nonstick skillet, heat 1 teaspoon of oil over medium-high heat until shimmering. Add the mushrooms. Cook, shaking the pan a few times, until the mushrooms are golden, 3 to 4 minutes. Stir in the spinach, and season with salt. Cook until just wilted, 1 to 2 minutes. Transfer the vegetables to a bowl. Stir in the parsley; set aside.

Heat the remaining teaspoon of oil in the same skillet. Season the eggs with salt and pour into the pan. Cook, without disturbing the eggs, until the edges are set. Using a rubber spatula, lift underneath the edges of the egg while tilting the pan so any uncooked egg can slide underneath and cook. Cover one half of the eggs with the vegetable mixture. Sprinkle the cheese on top. Fold the plain egg over the half with the vegetables, to create a half moon. Cook for 1 minute more. Serve immediately.

Calories 500   Fat 38   Protein 34   Carbs 5   Fiber 1   Net carbs 4

LUNCH

Bacon, Avocado & Turkey Lettuce Wraps

Spicy Sesame Zoodles

Italian Stuffed Peppers

Warm Spinach & Roast Chicken Salad with Bacon
Vinaigrette

Chicken Caesar Salad with Parmesan Crisps

Buffalo Chicken Wings with Ranch Dipping Sauce

Bacon & Shrimp Lollipops

Shrimp & Avocado Cobb Salad

Pork-Fried Cauliflower Couscous

Bacon, Avocado & Turkey Lettuce Wraps

Serves: 2

Cooking up a batch of bacon and keeping it in the fridge makes for fast weekday lunches. A quick reheat in a skillet is enough to crisp it up. Feel free to swap in leftover roast chicken in place of turkey.

- 2 leaves curly kale
- 1 tablespoon mayonnaise
- 4 slices cooked bacon
- 1 avocado, pitted & sliced
- 4 slices turkey

Lay each leaf of kale on a cutting board. Brush with the mayonnaise. On half of each leaf, layer two pieces of bacon, half the avocado slices, and two slices of turkey. Roll up starting with the end that's filled. Enjoy.

Calories 510   Fat 44   Protein 17   Carbs 14.6   Fiber 7.3   Net carbs 7.3

Spicy Sesame Zoodles

Serves: 2

Cold sesame noodles used to be a favorite lunch of mine. Here I'm swapping in zucchini noodles (Zoodles, page 99). The sauce traditionally has a sweetener to balance out the heaviness of the almond butter. I've opted to leave it out here, but if you prefer, you can add ½ packet of stevia to the dressing as you whisk it together in the bowl.

- ½ lime
- ¼ cup creamy almond butter
- 1 tablespoon soy sauce
- 1 tablespoon sesame oil
- ½ teaspoon red pepper chili flakes
- Sea salt to taste
- ½ cup shredded red cabbage
- Handful of fresh cilantro, leaves and stems chopped
- 2 scallions, chopped
- ⅓ cup sliced almonds
- Zoodles (page 99)

Juice the lime into a deep bowl.

Add the almond butter, soy sauce, sesame oil, and chili flakes to the bowl. Season with salt. Whisk until well blended.

Add the cabbage, cilantro, scallions, almonds, and Zoodles to the bowl. Toss to coat. Serve immediately, or chill before serving.

Calories 507   Fat 47.6   Protein 12.9   Carbs 14   Fiber 6.8   Net carbs 7.2

ITALIAN STUFFED PEPPERS

Serves: 2

- 1 tablespoon extra virgin olive oil
- 8 ounces ground beef
- Sea salt and freshly ground black pepper
- 1 garlic clove, chopped
- 1 cup Slow-Simmered Tomato Sauce (page 94)
- ½ teaspoon dried basil
- ½ teaspoon dried oregano
- 1 cup Cauliflower Couscous (page 98)
- 4 ounces shredded mozzarella
- 2 red bell peppers

In a medium skillet, add the oil and heat until shimmering. Add the beef and use a fork to break up any chunks (you want little bits of meat). Season with salt and pepper. Cook until well browned. Use slotted spoon to transfer to a bowl; set aside.

Add the garlic to the pan. Sauté until fragrant, about 1 minute.

Stir in the tomato sauce, basil, and oregano, and add the meat back to the pan. Season with salt and pepper. Reduce heat to low, and simmer for 5 minutes.

Preheat the oven to 375°F.

Remove the meat filling from the heat and let cool slightly while the oven preheats.

Stir the Cauliflower Couscous and half the mozzarella into the filling.

Slice the tops off the bell peppers and scoop out the seeds. Evenly spoon the meat filling into the peppers. Arrange the peppers in an 8-inch loaf pan. Sprinkle the remaining mozzarella on top.

Bake 35 to 40 minutes, until the peppers are soft and the cheese is lightly golden. Serve hot.

Calories 574   Fat 40.2   Protein 36.8   Carbs 17.9   Fiber 4.2   Net carbs 13.7

WARM SPINACH & ROAST CHICKEN SALAD WITH BACON VINAIGRETTE

Serves: 2

Most people add cold bacon to a hot pan and then duck for cover from the splatter. The easiest way to avoid that is to add cold bacon to a *cold* pan (genius, right?). The drippings form the base for a flavorful dressing for what might otherwise seem a very simple salad. Leftover chicken from making the Bone Broth on page 90 or the Smoky Butter Roasted Chicken on page 72 both work well here.

- 4 slices bacon
- 1 garlic clove, smashed
- 2 teaspoons Dijon mustard
- 2 tablespoons red wine vinegar
- Salt
- Freshly ground black pepper
- 2 cups cubed or shredded cooked chicken
- 4 cups packed baby spinach

Add the bacon to a cold 8-inch skillet, and place over medium-high heat. Cook until crisp all over, turning once. Transfer to a paper-towel-lined plate.

In the same pan, add the garlic. Sauté until fragrant, about 1 minute. Discard the garlic. Off the heat, whisk in the mustard and vinegar. Season with salt and pepper. Return skillet to a low flame. Stir in the chicken, and cook until warmed, 1 to 2 minutes. Remove pan from the heat, stir in the spinach, then immediately divide the salad between two shallow bowls. Enjoy immediately.

Calories 489   Fat 32   Protein 43.8   Carbs 2.9   Fiber 1.3   Net carbs 1.6

Chicken Caesar Salad with Parmesan Crisps

Serves: 2

This salad is a favorite for a few reasons. First, it uses up leftover roast chicken from the recipe on page 72. If you're craving it but don't have leftover roast chicken, you can use store-bought rotisserie chicken (stick to the herb- or plain-roasted ones, since they probably won't have any added sugars). It's also an easy lunch to pack for busy weekdays.

- ¼ cup mayonnaise
- 1 garlic clove
- 1 teaspoon freshly squeezed lemon juice
- ¼ teaspoon soy sauce
- ½ teaspoon anchovy paste
- 1 tablespoon Parmesan cheese
- ¼ teaspoon Dijon mustard
- 1 bunch romaine hearts, chopped
- 2 cups leftover Smoky Butter Roasted Chicken
- 6 Parmesan Crisps (page 97)

To make the dressing, add the mayonnaise, garlic, lemon juice, soy sauce, anchovy paste, Parmesan, and mustard to a blender. Blend until the dressing is smooth and creamy.

In a deep bowl, combine the lettuce and chicken. Add half of the dressing and toss until well coated. Garnish with Parmesan Crisps. Serve immediately.

Calories 321   Fat 29   Protein 12.4   Carbs 2.8   Fiber 1   Net carbs 1.8

BUFFALO CHICKEN WINGS WITH RANCH DIPPING SAUCE

Serves: 2

- 1 teaspoon baking powder
- ½ teaspoon garlic powder
- ½ teaspoon black pepper, plus more as needed
- ¼ teaspoon sea salt, plus more as needed
- 8 chicken wings (wing and drum)
- 2 tablespoons melted butter
- ¼ cup hot sauce (preferably one without added sugars)
- ¼ cup Homemade Ranch Dressing (page 95)

Preheat the oven to 375°F. Generously brush an 11-by-17-inch baking sheet with olive oil.

Combine the baking powder, garlic powder, pepper, salt, and 1 tablespoon water in a deep bowl. Add the chicken and toss until well coated. Arrange the chicken in a single layer on the prepared pan. Bake for 20 to 25 minutes, turning halfway through, until golden on both sides.

Meanwhile, whisk together the butter and hot sauce in a small bowl. Pour over the chicken, stirring to make sure it's well coated. Increase the oven temperature to 400°F. Bake 10 to 15 minutes more, turning halfway through, until crispy.

Serve the chicken wings hot with the Homemade Ranch Dressing.

Calories 310   Fat 26.3   Protein 16.3   Carbs 2.4   Fiber 0.1   Net carbs 2.3

Bacon & Shrimp Lollipops

Serves: 2

This play on surf and turf is perfect party food, so keep this recipe in your back pocket for when you're hosting or going to a friend's house.

- 6 pieces bacon (thin-cut works best)
- 6 jumbo shrimp, shelled and deveined
- 2 wooden or metal skewers

If using wooden skewers, soak them in water for 2 hours to avoid any splinters.

Preheat the broiler of your oven.

Use one piece of bacon to wrap around one shrimp (imagine you're looping a piece of ribbon around a ring) to cover it completely. Repeat with the remaining bacon and shrimp.

Add three pieces to each skewer, sliding the skewer through the shrimp lengthwise (instead of right through the center). Place on a rimmed sheet pan.

Broil 4 to 5 minutes, until browned. Turn and broil 4 to 5 minutes more until cooked through. Serve hot.

Calories 410   Fat 34   Protein 25   Carbs 1   Fiber 0   Net carbs 1

Shrimp & Avocado Cobb Salad

Serves: 2

- 8 large shrimp, peeled and deveined
- 1 head Boston lettuce, chopped
- 1 romaine heart, chopped
- 10 grape tomatoes, halved
- 4 hard-boiled eggs, cut in half
- 4 slices cooked bacon, crumbled
- 1 avocado, pitted and chopped
- ¼ cup Easy Homemade Vinaigrette (page 96)

To cook the shrimp, fill a 2-quart pot with water and bring to a boil over high heat. Add the shrimp. Cover and remove the pot from heat. Set aside for 10 minutes. Drain the shrimp and set them in a bowl of ice water to stop the cooking process; set aside.

Arrange the lettuces, tomatoes, eggs, bacon, avocado, and shrimp between two shallow bowls. Drizzle the dressing on top. Serve immediately.

> My method for making foolproof hard-boiled eggs is to place the eggs in a small pot filled with enough water to cover them. Bring it to a boil over high heat. Remove from the heat, cover with a lid, and let sit for 10 minutes. Drain the water and set the eggs in a bowl of cold water to stop the cooking process. I find they're easier to peel when made a day or two in advance.

Calories 838   Fat 69.6   Protein 40   Carbs 17.9   Fiber 9.5   Net carbs 8.4

PORK-FRIED CAULIFLOWER COUSCOUS

Serves: 2

This is a great way to use up extra Cauliflower Couscous (page 98). In fact, it's a great reason to make the Cauliflower Couscous, so you can reap the rewards of leftovers — just be sure to make it at least a day in advance, since it needs to be cold to work best in this dish.

- 2 teaspoons olive oil
- 2 eggs, beaten
- Sea salt and freshly ground black pepper
- 2 boneless pork chops, diced
- 1 tablespoon sesame oil
- 1 teaspoon freshly grated ginger
- 1 garlic clove, chopped fine
- 3 cups cold, cooked Cauliflower Couscous
- 3 tablespoons soy sauce
- 2 to 3 scallions, chopped

Heat 1 teaspoon of the olive oil in a deep skillet over medium-high heat until shimmering. Add the eggs, and cook, stirring, until cooked through, about 1 minute. Transfer to a small bowl.

Increase the heat to high, and add another teaspoon of olive oil to the pan. Add the pork, and sauté until golden and cooked through, 2 to 3 minutes. Transfer to the bowl with the eggs.

Heat the sesame oil in the same skillet. Add the ginger and garlic. Sauté until fragrant, 15 to 30 seconds. Add the Cauliflower Couscous, making sure to break up any clumps. Stir in the soy sauce and scallions. Add the pork and egg back to the pan. Sauté until the Cauliflower Couscous is heated through, 1 to 2 minutes. Serve hot.

Calories 342   Fat 29.5   Protein 16.6   Carbs 5.8   Fiber 1.1   Net carbs 4.7

DINNER

Kimchi Pork Lettuce Cups

Thai Turkey Burgers

BBQ Flank Steak and Cabbage Slaw

Beef Bolognese

Smoky Butter Roasted Chicken

Sheet-Pan Chicken Fajita Bowls

Almond-Crusted Salmon Patties

Swedish Meatballs

Magic Keto Pizza

KIMCHI PORK LETTUCE CUPS

Serves: 2

This Thai-inspired dish packs a punch of flavor. To eat it, scoop up some of the pork filling with a lettuce leaf, roll it up, and dig in. For a different twist, you can nix the lettuce and serve the filling tossed with zoodles.

- 2 teaspoons extra virgin olive oil
- 1 garlic clove, chopped fine
- 8 ounces ground pork
- Handful of fresh cilantro, chopped
- ½ cup kimchi, chopped fine
- 1 teaspoon fish sauce (Red Boat fish sauce has no added sugar)
- 1½ teaspoons soy sauce
- Sea salt to taste
- 1 small head Boston lettuce, leaves removed, rinsed and patted dry
- Lime wedges, for garnish
- Fresh mint, for garnish

In a 10-inch skillet, heat the oil over medium-high heat until shimmering. Add the garlic, and sauté until lightly golden, 1 to 2 minutes. Add the pork, using a fork to break up any large chunks. Add the cilantro, kimchi, fish sauce, and soy sauce. Season with salt. Reduce heat to medium-low. Continue cooking, stirring every couple of minutes, until the pork is completely cooked through, 7 to 9 minutes.

Meanwhile, arrange the lettuce leaves on a platter.

Spoon the cooked pork filling over the lettuce leaves. Garnish with lime wedges and fresh mint. Serve immediately.

Calories 322   Fat 24.3   Protein 19.7   Carbs 6.8   Fiber 2.6   Net carbs 4.2

THAI TURKEY BURGERS

Serves: 2

These burgers pack a punch of flavor, in all the good ways. If you've got some carbs to spare and are really craving a bun for them, make the Easy Keto Bread on page 92 to serve them on. The Zucchini Fries on page 100 are a must!

- 12 ounces ground turkey
- 1 garlic clove
- 1 teaspoon fresh grated ginger
- Handful of fresh cilantro, stems and leaves chopped fine
- 2 teaspoons red curry paste
- ½ teaspoon sea salt, plus more to taste
- 4 teaspoons mayonnaise
- ½ teaspoon Dijon mustard
- 2 teaspoons extra virgin olive oil
- Freshly ground black pepper
- 2 romaine heart leaves or curly kale leaves

In a medium bowl, add the turkey, garlic, ginger, half of the chopped cilantro, chili paste, and salt. Mix well. Divide the mixture into 2 equal portions, and shape into flat 4-inch patties.

In a small bowl, mix together the mayonnaise, Dijon, and remaining cilantro. Season with salt and pepper.

Heat the oil in a medium skillet over medium–high heat. Add the burgers, and cook until browned underneath, 4 to 5 minutes. Flip, and continue cooking until browned on the other side and cooked through, 4 to 5 minutes more.

Wrap each burger in a lettuce leaf to serve.

Calories 451   Fat 29   Protein 45.5   Carbs 1.8   Fiber 0.8   Net carbs 1

BBQ Flank Steak & Cabbage Slaw

Serves: 4

Butter may sound like an odd addition to BBQ sauce, but it creates a thick, rich-bodied sauce and adds extra fat to a particularly lean cut of meat.

- ¼ cup ketchup (a no-sugar-added variety, such as Primal Kitchen)
- 2 tablespoons butter, melted
- 1 teaspoon Dijon mustard
- ½ teaspoon onion powder
- ½ teaspoon Worcestershire sauce
- ½ teaspoon freshly ground black pepper, plus more as needed
- Sea salt to taste
- 1½ pounds flank steak
- ¼ cup mayonnaise
- 1 tablespoon apple cider vinegar
- ¼ teaspoon celery seed
- 2 cups shredded cabbage

Preheat the broiler in your oven to high with the rack positioned under the broiler plate.

In a small bowl, whisk together the ketchup, butter, mustard, onion powder, Worcestershire sauce, and black pepper to blend.

Place the steak on a rimmed sheet pan. Brush the sauce all over, top and bottom. Cook 5 to 7 minutes, until nicely browned on top. Turn, and cook 5 to 7 minutes more, to desired doneness. Let rest 5 minutes.

Meanwhile, prepare the slaw. In a small bowl, whisk together the mayonnaise, vinegar, and celery seed in a deep bowl. Season with salt and pepper. Add the cabbage and stir until well mixed. Set aside in the fridge. This may be prepared 1 day in advance.

Slice the steak, cutting against the grain, and serve with slaw.

Note: If you're planning ahead, you can marinate the steak 1 to 2 days in advance by placing it in a zip-top bag with the sauce in the fridge. Cook as directed.

Calories 392   Fat 25   Protein 37   Carbs 3   Fiber 1   Net carbs 2

BEEF BOLOGNESE

Serves: 4

Pasta is one thing many miss when first starting keto. Here the sauce gets all the attention, and once you taste a spoonful you'll know it's for good reason. It's perfect served over zoodles, but you can also go for an Italian sloppy Joe and serve it on Easy Keto Bread (page 92).

- 4 slices thick-cut bacon, chopped
- 1½ pounds ground beef
- Sea salt and freshly ground black pepper
- ¾ cup heavy cream
- 1 can (28 ounces) tomato purée
- Zoodles, to serve (page 99)
- Grated Parmesan cheese, to serve (optional)

Add the bacon to a cold deep skillet, and place over medium-high heat. Cook until crisp all over, turning once. Transfer to a bowl using a slotted spoon.

Crumble the beef into the skillet. Season with salt and pepper. Cook, stirring occasionally, until well browned, 5 to 7 minutes.

Reduce the heat to medium–low. Stir in the cream. Cook, stirring occasionally, until the cream is mostly evaporated but the meat isn't dry, about 10 minutes.

Stir in the tomato purée, making sure to scrape up any browned bits from the bottom of the pan. Season with salt. Bring to a boil. Reduce heat to low. Cook for 2 to 3 hours, stirring occasionally (see Note). Add a few tablespoons of water, as needed, to prevent the sauce from sticking to the pan.

About 30 minutes before the sauce is ready, begin preparing the Zoodles on page 99.

Serve the Bolognese over the zoodles, with Pecorino, if desired.

Note: Once you add the tomato purée to the pan, you can transfer the sauce to a slow cooker, and cook on low for 4 to 6 hours.

Calories 532   Fat 36.2   Protein 42.6   Carbs 8.4   Fiber 3.7   Net carbs 3.7

SMOKY BUTTER ROASTED CHICKEN

Serves: 4

Two things to know when making the perfect roast chicken: high heat is your friend, and you don't need to truss the chicken (tie the legs and wings back). Sure, trussing looks pretty, but leaving the chicken as is allows the heat to circulate throughout, helping it cook faster and evenly. For a simpler version of this recipe, omit the paprika, garlic, and herbs from the butter.

- 6 tablespoons butter, softened
- 1½ teaspoons smoked paprika
- 1 garlic clove, grated
- Handful of fresh flat-leaf parsley, chopped
- Sea salt and freshly ground black pepper to taste
- 3½-pound whole chicken

Preheat the oven to 450°F.

In a small bowl, combine the butter, paprika, garlic, parsley, salt, and pepper. Using a fork, mix together until well blended.

Place the chicken in a roasting pan. Rub the butter mixture all over. Cook for 20 minutes, then add 1/2 cup of water to the bottom of the pan—this helps prevent the drippings from smoking, while making a natural sauce from the juices. Roast for 40 to 50 minutes more, basting every 15 minutes, until the juices run clear and an instant-read thermometer inserted in the thigh registers 165°F.

Remove the chicken from the oven and let sit for 5 to 10 minutes before carving.

Calories 614   Fat 51   Protein 37   Carbs 0.5   Fiber 0   Net carbs 0.5

SHEET-PAN CHICKEN FAJITA BOWLS

Serves: 2

- 2 chicken thighs, skin-on
- 2 chicken legs, skin-on
- 2 to 3 tablespoons butter, softened
- 1 teaspoon taco seasoning (be sure to choose one without hidden sweeteners)
- Sea salt and freshly ground black pepper
- 1 poblano pepper, seeded and sliced
- 2 garlic cloves, chopped
- 1 tablespoon extra virgin olive oil
- Cauliflower Couscous (page 98)
- 1 lime, zested and remaining lime cut in quarters
- Small bunch fresh cilantro, leaves and stems chopped

Preheat the oven to 450°F.

Rub the chicken pieces all over with 1 to 2 tablespoons of butter. Place in a single layer on a 9-by-13-inch rimmed baking sheet. Sprinkle with the taco seasoning; season with salt and pepper. Add the poblano and garlic to the pan, and drizzle with the olive oil.

Roast until chicken begins to brown, 15 to 20 minutes. Give the peppers a stir to coat with the pan juices. Add a few tablespoons of water if the pan seems too dry. Spoon some of the juices over the chicken. Bake for 15 to 20 minutes more, until chicken reaches 165°F when tested with an instant-read thermometer.

Meanwhile, prepare the Cauliflower Couscous as directed

on page 98. Once cooked, stir in the lime zest and half the cilantro.

To serve, divide the couscous between two wide, shallow bowls. Top each with a chicken leg and thigh, then some of the peppers. Spoon some of the pan juices on top. Sprinkle with remaining cilantro and enjoy!

Calories 455   Fat 32   Protein 36.3   Carbs 6   Fiber 2.3   Net carbs 3.7

ALMOND-CRUSTED SALMON PATTIES

Serves: 4

Some people notice an uptick in their grocery bills when switching to keto. Using canned salmon gives you more bang for your buck, while you still get the benefits of omega-3 plus a boost of calcium.

- 2 cans (6 ounces) wild pink salmon
- 1 tablespoon Dijon mustard
- ¼ teaspoon paprika
- Handful of fresh flat-leaf parsley, chopped
- 1 large egg
- Sea salt and freshly ground black pepper to taste
- 1 cup almond meal
- 2 tablespoons coconut oil

In the bowl of a food processor, combine the salmon, mustard, paprika, parsley, egg, salt, pepper, and ½ cup of the almond meal. Pulse the mixture until it is coarsely blended (a few chunks of salmon remaining). Transfer to a bowl, cover, and chill in the fridge for at least 1 hour, or overnight.

When ready to cook, divide the salmon mixture into 8 even balls. Flatten them into patties. Use the remaining ½ cup of almond meal to coat them all over.

In a 10-inch nonstick skillet, melt 1 tablespoon of the coconut oil over medium heat until shimmering. Add the patties to the pan (you might need to do this in batches, so as to not overcrowd the pan). Cook until golden underneath, 3 to 4 minutes. Turn, and cook until golden on the other side, 3 to 4 minutes more. Serve hot.

Calories 369   Fat 26   Protein 26   Carbs 7   Fiber 3.5   Net carbs 3.5

Swedish Meatballs

Serves: 2

- 1 pound ground beef
- 1 egg
- 1 garlic clove, grated
- ¼ teaspoon fresh grated nutmeg
- 2 tablespoons chopped fresh flat-leaf parsley
- ¼ cup almond flour
- ½ teaspoon sea salt
- Fresh ground black pepper to taste
- 2 tablespoons butter
- 1 tablespoon Dijon mustard (be sure to buy one without added sugars)
- 1 teaspoon soy sauce
- 2 teaspoons coconut flour
- ¾ cup chicken or beef broth
- ½ cup heavy cream

In a medium bowl, add the beef, egg, garlic, nutmeg, parsley, almond flour, salt, and pepper. Stir together with your hands, or a wooden spoon if that's more comfortable, until well mixed. Shape into 8 balls.

Melt the butter in an 8-inch skillet over medium-high heat. Add the meatballs. Cook until browned all over, turning as needed, 8 to 10 minutes. Transfer to a dish; set aside.

Discard all but 1 tablespoon of the fat from the skillet. Over medium heat, stir in the mustard, soy sauce, and coconut flour, scraping up any browned bits. Stir in the broth. Bring to a boil. Reduce heat to a simmer and stir in the cream. Season with salt and pepper. Add the meatballs back to the pan, and cook 8 to 10 minutes more, until sauce thickens. Serve hot.

Calories 728   Fat 51   Protein 59.6   Carbs 8.4   Fiber 2.8   Net carbs 5.6

MAGIC KETO PIZZA

Serves: 2 to 4

Pizza is one food lots of people miss when cutting out carbs. As an Italian girl from Brooklyn, I understand this very well, and I am really excited to share this recipe. Let's be real: nothing will ever compare with a traditional crust, but this crust is truly amazing, even magical. The real test is when you hold up a slice that defies gravity and it doesn't flop over! The only thing you're left to ponder as you devour it is whether to fold or not fold.

FOR THE CRUST

- 1 egg
- 6 ounces shredded mozzarella cheese
- 4 tablespoons butter, softened and broken into chunks
- ½ cup superfine, blanched almond flour
- 6 tablespoons coconut flour
- 2 teaspoons baking powder
- ¼ teaspoon sea salt

FOR THE PIZZA

- ¾ cup Slow-Simmered Tomato Sauce (page 94)
- 6 ounces shredded mozzarella cheese
- Any desired keto-friendly toppings

Preheat the oven to 375°F.

To make the crust, add the egg, mozzarella, butter, flours, baking powder, and sea salt to the bowl of a food processor. Pulse until it forms a rough ball. Very lightly dust a counter with coconut flour. Knead the dough until it becomes smooth, 30 to 60 seconds, adding more coconut flour only as needed to keep the dough from sticking.

Place the dough on a sheet of parchment paper. Cover with another sheet of parchment or waxed paper. Roll into a 1/8-inch-thick circle. Remove the top layer of parchment. Slide crust, still on the parchment paper, onto a pizza pan. Bake until lightly golden, about 15 minutes.

Spread the tomato sauce on top, leaving a ¼- to ½-inch border at the edge. Sprinkle with the remaining mozzarella cheese and add any desired toppings. Bake until cheese is melted and bubbling, and crust is crispy, 15 to 20 minutes more. Let rest for 2 minutes before slicing and serving.

To heat leftovers, add the slices to a nonstick skillet over medium heat. Cook until hot, and enjoy.

Calories 169   Fat 10   Protein 16   Carbs 5.4   Fiber 2   Net carbs 3.4

Nutritional analysis is per slice.

TREATS & BEVERAGES

Orange Espresso Chia Pudding

Almond Butter Cup Fat Bombs

Almond Joy Avocado Mousse

Berry Cheesecake Bars

Coconut Whipped Cream

Mocha Bulletproof Coffee

Bulletproof Coconut Chai

Orange Espresso Chia Pudding

Serves: 2

I'm convinced there's a chia-pudding conspiracy out there. Every recipe says it should be chilled overnight. I've never had success with this method, as chia seeds really need a full 24 hours to properly absorb the liquids and plump up. So plan ahead when making these. The good news is the recipe can be doubled, and it keeps a few days in the fridge. Make a batch if you like, and enjoy chia pudding all week long.

Fun Fact: Oranges aren't allowed on keto, but you can use the zest with abandon since all the sugar is in the fruit itself.

- ¾ cup unsweetened almond milk
- 2 tablespoons espresso or strongly brewed coffee
- Zest of 1 orange
- 1 packet stevia powder (optional)
- 4 tablespoons white chia seeds
- 2 tablespoons sliced almonds, toasted

In a small bowl, whisk together the coconut milk, espresso, orange zest, and stevia, if using. Stir in the chia seeds until well mixed.

Divide between two 8-ounce mason jars. Cover with the lid. Chill for at least 24 hours, and up to 2 days. The pudding will keep, covered, for up to 4 days. To serve, top each pudding with half the almonds.

Calories 206   Fat 14.4   Protein 7.2   Carbs 14.9   Fiber 10.1   Net carbs 4.8

Chocolate Almond Butter Cup Fat Bombs

Makes: 12 bite-sized pieces (serving size 1 piece)

- 6 tablespoons dark chocolate chips (Lily's are sweetened with stevia)
- 6 tablespoons almond butter
- 6 tablespoons coconut oil
- 1 packet stevia powder

Line a 12-cup mini muffin tin with paper liners.

In a small microwave-safe bowl, melt the chocolate chips in 30-second intervals. Pour half into the prepared tin cups. Let cool for 5 minutes.

In a small pot, combine the almond butter and coconut oil over low heat. Cook until melted, stirring together to mix. Stir in the stevia. Pour an even amount over the chocolate in the paper liners.

Evenly pour the remaining chocolate over the almond-butter filling. Set in the fridge to firm up, at least two hours. Keep refrigerated.

Calories 135   Fat 13.4   Protein 2.2   Carbs 6   Fiber 2.8   Net carbs 3.2

ALMOND JOY AVOCADO MOUSSE

Serves: 2

One of my favorite candy bars in keto dessert form!

- 1 ripe avocado, pitted and fruit scooped from skin
- 1 to 2 packets stevia powder
- 2 tablespoons cocoa powder
- ½ teaspoon vanilla extract
- 6 to 8 tablespoons coconut milk (depends on size of avocado)
- 1 tablespoon dark chocolate chips
- 1 tablespoon coconut flakes
- 1 tablespoon sliced almonds
- Coconut Whipped Cream, to serve (optional; page 86)

Add the avocado, stevia, cocoa powder, vanilla, and coconut milk to the bowl of a food processor.

Pulse until smooth.

Evenly spoon the pudding into 2 small bowls or jars. Top evenly with the chocolate chips, coconut flakes, and almonds. Cover with plastic film, and chill for at least 2 hours, until pudding is set. May be made up to 1 day in advance. Top with Coconut Whipped Cream before serving, if using.

Calories 268   Fat 37   Protein 263.4   Carbs 22.7   Fiber 13   Net carbs 9.7

BERRY CHEESECAKE BARS

Makes: 8 bars (serving size 1 bar)

FOR THE CRUST

- 3 tablespoons butter, melted
- 1 cup almond flour
- 1 packet stevia powder

FOR THE FILLING

- 8 ounces full-fat cream cheese, softened
- 1 egg
- 2 packets stevia powder
- 1 teaspoon lemon juice
- ¼ cup raspberries or blueberries

Preheat the oven to 350°F.

Line an 8-inch loaf pan with a piece of parchment paper long enough to hang over the sides (this acts as a sling to lift the bars out when done).

To make the crust, combine the butter, almond flour, and stevia in a small bowl. Stir with until mixed, then press into bottom of the prepared baking pan. Bake until set, 7 to 8 minutes. Let cool completely.

To make the filling, combine the cream cheese, egg, stevia, and lemon juice in a medium bowl. Stir with a fork until well blended. Pour over the crust.

Mash the berries lightly with the back of a fork, just to break them up a bit. Scatter over the filling and use a butter knife to swirl them through the cream–cheese mixture.

Bake 15 to 20 minutes, until center is mostly set (it'll jiggle slightly like Jell-O). Let cool completely, then chill for at least three hours, or overnight, before cutting into 8 even bars.

Calories 229   Fat 21.7   Protein 5.6   Carbs 5.7   Fiber 1.6   Net carbs 4.1

Coconut Whipped Cream

Makes: 1 cup (serving size 1 tablespoon)

Making a keto-friendly whipped cream at home is easier than you think! All it requires is advance planning, since the canned coconut milk needs to be chilled for a full day in order for it to whip properly. It's perfect as a topping for the Almond Joy Avocado Mousse on page 83, or just add some berries and enjoy it as a quick snack. Want to jazz it up? Try adding a dash of cinnamon, 1 teaspoon of cocoa, or some citrus zest before you whip it.

- 1 can (15 ounces) full-fat, unsweetened coconut milk

24 hours before you plan to make this whipped cream, place the can of coconut milk in the fridge.

The next day, open the can, scoop out the solids and add them to a small bowl (save the remaining coconut water for another use). Using a handheld mixer, whip the coconut solids until fluffy and thickened into a slightly stiff cream. Use immediately.

Calories 61   Fat 6.3   Protein 0.6   Carbs 1.4   Fiber 0.6   Net carbs 0.8

Mocha Bulletproof Coffee

Serves: 1

When you need a quick boost of energy that also leaves you feeling full, bulletproof coffee is the way to go. The butter and MCT oil bulk it up into a satisfying mini-meal. It's a great way to start the day or as an afternoon pick-me-up to keep snacking at bay. Should you want a little sweet touch, you can add ½ packet stevia powder—any more will accentuate coffee's natural bitter notes.

- ¾ cup hot brewed coffee
- 2 tablespoons butter
- 1 tablespoon MCT oil (optional)
- ½ teaspoon cocoa powder
- ¼ teaspoon cinnamon

Add all the ingredients to a blender bowl. Blend on high for 30 to 60 seconds, until frothy.

Calories 327   Fat 39.4   Protein 0.7   Carbs 0   Fiber 0   Net carbs 0

BULLETPROOF COCONUT CHAI

Serves: 1

Traditional chai is loaded with sugar. This version, a tea relative of the popular bulletproof coffee, delivers all the aromatic flavors plus a boost of energy without providing the cloyingly sweet consequences.

- 12 ounces hot brewed black tea
- 2 tablespoons butter
- 1 tablespoon MCT oil
- ¼ cup unsweetened coconut milk
- ¼ teaspoon cardamom
- ¼ teaspoon fresh grated ginger
- ¼ teaspoon ground cloves
- ½ teaspoon cinnamon

Add all the ingredients to a blender bowl. Blend on high for 30 to 60 seconds, until frothy.

Calories 464   Fat 51   Protein 3.5   Carbs 7   Fiber 1   Net carbs 6

BASICS

Slow-Roasted Chicken-Bone Broth

Easy Keto Bread

Slow-Simmered Tomato Sauce

Homemade Ranch Dressing

Easy Homemade Vinaigrette

Homemade Parmesan Crisps

Cauliflower Couscous

Zoodles

Zucchini Fries

SLOW-ROASTED CHICKEN-BONE BROTH

Makes: about 1 quart

- 8 chicken thighs, skin-on and bone-in
- 3 garlic cloves, peeled and smashed
- 4 celery ribs, cut into 2-inch pieces
- Sea salt and freshly ground black pepper
- 3 tablespoons extra virgin olive oil
- Handful of fresh flat-leaf Italian parsley

Preheat your oven to 475°F, with the rack adjusted to the upper center position.

Arrange the chicken pieces, garlic, and celery in a 9-by-13-inch roasting pan. Season with salt and pepper. Roast for 15 minutes.

Drizzle the oil on top. Roast for 15 more minutes.

Add the parsley and pour 6 cups of water into the pan. Roast for 30 more minutes.

Reduce the oven temperature to 275°F. Roast for at least 3 hours and up to 6 hours, adding more water to the pan as needed to keep the chicken covered by about two-thirds. You want the tops to get nicely browned but remain mostly submerged so the meat braises. Taste the broth as it cooks, and add more salt, as needed, according to your tastes.

Using a slotted spoon, transfer the chicken to a plate. Once cooled, remove the meat, and discard the bones. The chicken is perfect as a simple sandwich on Easy Keto Bread (page 92)—don't forget the mayo! It can also be used in the Cobb Salad on page 63 instead of salmon, or the Chicken Caesar Salad on page 60.

Strain the stock, discarding any solids. Let the stock cool completely, then pack in containers, and refrigerate for up to 1 week, or store in the freezer for up to 2 months.

Calories 40   Fat 0.3   Protein 9.4   Carbs 0.6   Fiber 0   Net carbs 0.6

Nutritional analysis is based on one cup.

Easy Keto Bread

Yes, bread really is possible on keto. Hello, avocado toast! Unlike so many of the bread recipes out there, this one doesn't taste eggy. I really love the microwave version, but I am including an option to bake them too. The baked version is lighter in texture, and it must cool completely before you use it, or it'll crumble. The microwave bread is *perfect* for slicing and toasting when you want bread in less than 2 minutes (no joke). The texture reminds me of crumpets with all the nooks and crannies, and it is lovely split and toasted in a skillet with some butter (a conventional toaster works too).

Note: The smaller size is great for sliders, while the larger makes a great burger bun.

- 2 tablespoons butter, melted
- 1 large egg
- 1 tablespoon water or almond milk
- 2 tablespoons almond flour
- 1 tablespoon coconut flour
- ½ teaspoon baking powder
- ⅛ teaspoon sea salt

MICROWAVE METHOD

Use a pastry brush to coat the sides and bottoms of two 3½-inch (6-ounce) or one 5-inch (10-ounce) microwave-safe ramekins with some of the butter.

In a small bowl, whisk together the egg and water or almond milk. Whisk in the flours, baking powder, and salt.

Cook on high for 60 to 90 seconds for small breads and 1 to 2 minutes for larger ones, until cooked through (cook small ramekins one at a time for best results). Test for doneness by gently tapping the center with your finger; if it springs back, that means it's cooked through. Let cool for 1 minute. Slide a knife around the inside rim to loosen the bread. Turn out onto a board. Slice in half and use as you would sandwich bread.

OVEN METHOD

Preheat the oven to 400°F. Cut out parchment circles to line the bottom of two 3½-inch (6-ounce) or one 5-inch (10-ounce) oven-safe ramekin. Generously grease the sides with butter.

In a small bowl, whisk together the egg and water or almond milk. Whisk in the flours, baking powder, and salt.

Scrape the batter into the prepared ramekin. Bake 12 to 18 minutes, until cooked through. Start checking smaller ones at 10 minutes (a skewer inserted in the center should come out clean—don't test too soon or you'll deflate the bread). Let cool *completely,* then slice in half, and use as you would sandwich bread.

Calories 194   Fat 18   Protein 5.5   Carbs 4.5   Fiber 2   Net carbs 2.5

Nutritional analysis based on one small bread.

Slow-Simmered Tomato Sauce

Makes: about 3½ cups (serving size ½ cup)

- 1 can (28 ounces) San Marzano Tomatoes, whole and peeled
- 3 garlic cloves, smashed
- ¼ cup extra virgin olive oil
- ½ teaspoon dried basil
- Salt to taste

Add the tomatoes to a blender, and purée until smooth. You can alternately just crush them with your hands into the skillet if you prefer a chunkier-style sauce.

Add the tomatoes, garlic, olive oil, basil, and salt to a deep skillet. Cook, *uncovered,* for 45 minutes on low heat setting. Around 15 to 20 minutes into the cooking time, it'll start simmering vigorously — don't worry, that's what it should be doing.

After 45 minutes, the sauce is ready to serve, or you can transfer it to a jar, let cool completely, and store in fridge for up 3 days, or the freezer for up to 2 months.

Calories 88   Fat 8.3   Protein 1   Carbs 4.3   Fiber 2.2   Net carbs 2.1

Homemade Ranch Dressing

Makes: 1 cup (serving size 1 tablespoon)

- ½ cup mayonnaise
- ½ cup sour cream
- 2 teaspoons fresh squeezed lemon juice
- 1 teaspoon apple cider vinegar
- Handful of fresh chives, chopped

Whisk together the mayonnaise, sour cream, lemon juice, and vinegar with 2 tablespoons of water in a medium bowl. Stir in the chives. Season with salt and pepper. Refrigerate for up to 1 week. Shake well before each use.

Calories 60   Fat 6.2   Protein 0.6   Carbs 0.6   Fiber 0   Net carbs 0.6

Easy Homemade Vinaigrette

Makes: ¾ cup (serving size 1 tablespoon)

It happens. We all get busy, and some mornings it's impossible to pack a lunch. Keep a stash of this homemade dressing in your desk drawer, and you can always pull a keto-friendly lunch together from the salad bar. Stick to plain items, raw or steamed to ensure there are no hidden sweeteners, and grab a few hard-boiled eggs to bulk it up with fat and protein. (Don't worry about the herbs spoiling at room temperature—there's enough vinegar in the dressing to preserve them.)

- ½ cup extra virgin olive oil
- ¼ cup red wine vinegar
- 2 teaspoons whole-grain mustard
- Fresh chopped herbs of your choice (chives, cilantro, parsley, scallions)
- Sea salt and freshly ground black pepper to taste

Add all the ingredients to a mason jar. Cover tightly. Shake until well blended. Will keep at room temperature for up to 1 month. Be sure to shake well before each use.

Calories 83   Fat 9.5   Protein 0.1   Carbs 0.1   Fiber 0   Net carbs 0.1

HOMEMADE PARMESAN CRISPS

Makes: 12

Satisfy your chips fix with these easy-to-make cheese crisps. All you need is one ingredient and less than 10 minutes. They double as amazing croutons in salad (see the Chicken Caesar Salad with Parmesan Crisps on page 60).

- 2 ounces finely grated Pecorino-Locatelli cheese

OVEN METHOD

Preheat the oven to 350°F. Line a sheet pan with a silicon mat or parchment paper.

Drop the cheese onto the sheet in 12 mounds (about 2 tablespoons each), leaving 1 inch between so they have room to spread.

Bake 5 to 7 minutes, until golden and bubbly. They'll be soft when they come out of the oven but crisp up within a few minutes of cooling.

STOVE-TOP METHOD

Heat a nonstick skillet over medium–low heat. Drop mounds of cheese into the skillet (about 2 tablespoons each). Cook until the cheese melts and gets golden around the edges, about 2 minutes. Use an offset spatula to loosen and flip them. Cook 1 to 2 minutes more. Transfer to a plate and let cool a few minutes to crisp up.

Calories 38   Fat 2.5   Protein 3.5   Carbs 0.3   Fiber 0   Net carbs 0.3

CAULIFLOWER COUSCOUS

Serves: 2

One taste and you'll wonder where this simple side has been your whole life. The key is to stir the cauliflower couscous constantly while it cooks to help the water evaporate as it releases from the cauliflower; otherwise it might steam and get mushy.

- Small head cauliflower, florets only (save stems for another use)
- 2 tablespoons butter
- Sea salt to taste

Place the florets in a food processor. Pulse until broken down into fine bits resembling couscous.

In a deep nonstick skillet, melt 1 tablespoon of the butter. Add the cauliflower and cook until tender, stirring constantly, 5 to 7 minutes. Stir in the remaining tablespoon of butter. Season with salt and pepper. Fluff with a fork before serving.

Calories 116   Fat 11.8   Protein 1.3   Carbs 2.6   Fiber 1.4   Net carbs 1.2

ZOODLES

Serves: 2

It might seem silly to have a recipe for zoodles alone, but there's more to making them than just spiralizing zucchini.

- 3 medium zucchini
- 2 tablespoons butter
- Sea salt to taste
- Special equipment: spiralizer

Spiralize the zucchini into thin noodles. Lay a clean kitchen towel on the counter. Spread zucchini strands on the towel, and sprinkle with a little salt. This helps draw out excess water. Pat the noodles dry.

In a deep skillet, melt the butter over medium heat. Add the zoodles. Sauté 1 minute. You want them to stay a little raw to retain their texture. They're ready to eat, to serve as a side, or to use in another dish, such as the Spicy Sesame Zoodles (page 56).

Calories 107   Fat 11.6   Protein 0.8   Carbs 0.8   Fiber 0.3   Net carbs 0.5

ZUCCHINI FRIES

Serves: 2

Thanks to low-carb zucchini, you don't have to say good-bye to fries!

- 1 medium zucchini
- 1 egg, beaten
- ½ cup Parmesan cheese, shredded fine

Preheat the oven to 425°F, with the rack in the lowest position. Line a rimmed baking sheet with parchment paper.

Trim the zucchini ends. Cut the zucchini in half lengthwise, then cut each half into ¼-inch-thick strips. Dip each piece of zucchini into the egg, shaking off any excess, then dip into the cheese. Arrange coated zucchini in a single layer on the prepared pan.

Bake 25 to 30 minutes, turning halfway through, until crisp and golden. Serve hot.

Calories 120   Fat 8   Protein 10.9   Carbs 1.1   Fiber 0.1   Net carbs 1

PART III

RESOURCES

MEAL PLANNER 1: MEALS FROM NOON TO 6PM ONLY

Use the following pages to plan what you are going to eat over the next 4 weeks.

DAY 1

Morning	KETO
Noon	KETO
Before 6pm	KETO

DAY 2

Morning	KETO
Noon	KETO
Before 6pm	KETO

DAY 3

Morning	KETO
Noon	KETO
Before 6pm	KETO

DAY 4

Morning	KETO
Noon	KETO
Before 6pm	KETO

DAY 5

Morning	KETO
Noon	KETO
Before 6pm	KETO

DAY 6

Morning	KETO
Noon	KETO
Before 6pm	KETO

DAY 7

Morning	KETO
Noon	KETO
Before 6pm	KETO

DAY 8

Morning	FAST
Noon	KETO
Midday Snack	KETO
Before 6pm	KETO

DAY 9

Morning	FAST
Noon	KETO
Midday Snack	KETO
Before 6pm	KETO

DAY 10

Morning	FAST
Noon	KETO
Midday Snack	KETO
Before 6pm	KETO

DAY 11

Morning	FAST
Noon	KETO
Midday Snack	KETO
Before 6pm	KETO

DAY 12

Morning	FAST
Noon	KETO
Midday Snack	KETO
Before 6pm	KETO

DAY 13

Morning	FAST
Noon	KETO
Midday Snack	KETO
Before 6pm	KETO

DAY 14

Morning	KETO
Noon	KETO
Midday Snack	None
Before 6pm	KETO

DAY 15

Morning	FAST
Noon	KETO
Midday Snack	KETO
Before 6pm	KETO

DAY 16

Morning	FAST
Noon	KETO
Midday Snack	KETO
Before 6pm	KETO

DAY 17

Morning	FAST
Noon	KETO
Midday Snack	KETO
Before 6pm	KETO

DAY 18

Morning	FAST
Noon	KETO
Midday Snack	KETO
Before 6pm	KETO

DAY 19

Morning	FAST
Noon	KETO
Midday Snack	KETO
Before 6pm	KETO

DAY 20

Morning	FAST
Noon	KETO
Midday Snack	KETO
Before 6pm	KETO

DAY 21

Morning	KETO
Noon	KETO
Midday Snack	None
Before 6pm	KETO

DAY 22

Morning	FAST
Noon	KETO
Midday Snack	KETO
Before 6pm	KETO

DAY 23

Morning	FAST
Noon	KETO
Midday Snack	KETO
Before 6pm	KETO

DAY 24

Morning	FAST
Noon	KETO
Midday Snack	KETO
Before 6pm	KETO

DAY 25

Morning	FAST
Noon	KETO
Midday Snack	KETO
Before 6pm	KETO

DAY 26

Morning	FAST
Noon	KETO
Midday Snack	KETO
Before 6pm	KETO

DAY 27

Morning	FAST
Noon	KETO
Midday Snack	KETO
Before 6pm	KETO

DAY 28

Morning	KETO
Noon	KETO
Midday Snack	None
Before 6pm	KETO

MEAL PLANNER 2: ALTERNATE INTERMITTENT FASTING

DAY 1

Morning	KETO
Noon	KETO
Before 6pm	KETO

DAY 2

Morning	KETO
Noon	KETO
Before 6pm	KETO

DAY 3

Morning	KETO
Noon	KETO
Before 6pm	KETO

DAY 4

Morning	KETO
Noon	KETO
Before 6pm	KETO

DAY 5

Morning	KETO
Noon	KETO
Before 6pm	KETO

DAY 6

Morning	KETO
Noon	KETO
Before 6pm	KETO

DAY 7

Morning	KETO
Noon	KETO
Before 6pm	KETO

DAY 8

Morning	KETO
Noon	KETO
Before 6pm	FAST

DAY 9

Morning	KETO
Noon	KETO
Before 6pm	FAST

DAY 10

Morning	FAST
Noon	KETO
Before 6pm	KETO

DAY 11

Morning	KETO
Noon	KETO
Before 6pm	FAST

DAY 12

Morning	FAST
Noon	KETO
Before 6pm	KETO

DAY 13

Morning	KETO
Noon	KETO
Before 6pm	KETO

DAY 14

Morning	KETO
Noon	KETO
Before 6pm	FAST

DAY 15

Morning	FAST
Noon	KETO
Before 6pm	KETO

DAY 16

Morning	KETO
Noon	KETO
Before 6pm	FAST

DAY 17

Morning	FAST
Noon	KETO
Before 6pm	KETO

DAY 18

Morning	KETO
Noon	KETO
Before 6pm	FAST

DAY 19

Morning	FAST
Noon	KETO
Before 6pm	KETO

DAY 20

Morning	KETO
Noon	KETO
Before 6pm	KETO

DAY 21

Morning	KETO
Noon	KETO
Before 6pm	FAST

DAY 22

Morning	FAST
Noon	KETO
Before 6pm	KETO

DAY 23

Morning	KETO
Noon	KETO
Before 6pm	FAST

DAY 24

Morning	FAST
Noon	KETO
Before 6pm	KETO

DAY 25

Morning	KETO
Noon	KETO
Before 6pm	FAST

DAY 26

Morning	FAST
Noon	KETO
Before 6pm	KETO

DAY 27

Morning	KETO
Noon	KETO
Before 6pm	KETO

DAY 28

Morning	KETO
Noon	KETO
Before 6pm	FAST

About the Author

Jennifer Perillo is a food writer and recipe developer who runs the blog *In Jennie's Kitchen,* which has been featured in *Food 52, Saveur, Fine Cooking, Serious Eats, Bon Appetit,* and Oprah.com. She has worked as the consulting food editor at *Working Mother* magazine and has contributed to a variety of print and online publications and food websites, including *Food Network, Relish, Food 52, Cuisinart, Parade,* and *Parenting.* She is the author of *Homemade with Love.*

CPSIA information can be obtained
at www.ICGtesting.com
Printed in the USA
BVHW030513260119
538724BV00003B/105/P

9 780316 456418